ADHD and Adults

How to live with, improve, and manage your ADHD or ADD as an adult

Copyright 2015

Table Of Contents

Introduction 1
Chapter 1: What is ADHD or ADD? 2
Chapter 2: Signs and Symptoms of Adult ADHD/ADD 4
Chapter 3: Causes and Diagnosis of Adult ADHD/ADD 11
Chapter 4: What are the Treatments for ADHD/ADD? 15
Chapter 5: Living with ADHD/ADD 21
Conclusion 28
Check Out My Other Books Here: 29

Introduction

I want to thank you and congratulate you for downloading the book, "ADHD and Adults".

This book contains helpful information about how you can manage your ADHD, as an adult.

The following book will shed some light on what ADHD/ADD is, and in particular how it effects adults. People often consider ADHD or ADD to be a children's condition, and do not realize that it also has an impact on adults.

You will soon learn the symptoms of adult ADHD, what effect the condition will have on a person's life, and a range of strategies to assist in managing and improving the condition.

This book will explain to you tips and techniques that will allow you to gain control over your ADHD, and work on improving it as you grow older!

Thanks again for downloading this book, I hope you enjoy it!

Chapter 1:
What is ADHD or ADD?

As an adult, life can be a difficult balancing act. However, if you begin to find yourself to be disorganized, perennially late to work or appointments, forgetful, and overwhelmed by the enormous responsibilities you have to face, then you might be suffering from adult ADHD/ADD. This condition is not just for children and affects many adults. The condition can have frustrating symptoms that hinder almost all aspects of life, from relationships to careers. But like ADHD in children, there is hope and help is available. The moment you understand the challenges you have to face, you can learn how to compensate for the areas that you are struggling with and further develop your strengths.

What is Adult ADHD/ADD?

Attention deficit hyperactivity disorder (ADHD), also known as attention deficit disorder (ADD), is a condition characterized by hyperactivity, impulsiveness, and inattention. Medical experts now know that about 60% of children diagnosed with ADHD will carry the symptoms to adulthood. This is about 4% of the adult population in the United States, or about 8 million adults. However, the real cause of concern is that only a few adults are diagnosed and/or treated for the condition.

Adults suffering from ADHD may find it difficult to follow even the simplest directions, remember information, concentrate on organization, and meet deadlines. If these difficulties are not managed and controlled appropriately, they might cause associated behavioral, social, emotional, academic, and vocational problems.

Common Behaviors Associated with Adult ADHD

The following may or may not be related to ADHD but these are identified to directly stem from it:

- Chronic boredom
- Anxiety
- Depression
- Chronic forgetfulness
- Impulsiveness
- Difficulty with anger management
- Low self-esteem
- Extreme mood swings
- Procrastination and poor organizational skills
- Low tolerance to disappointments and frustrations
- Relationship problems
- Drug addiction

These may manifest as mild to severe symptoms. Although with ADHD, a person's concentration is often limited, some adults will be able to concentrate extremely well at particular tasks, especially when they find these tasks interesting.

Chapter 2:
Signs and Symptoms of Adult ADHD/ADD

Adults with ADHD/ADD manifest different symptoms from children suffering from the condition. The symptoms are unique for every person suffering from ADHD/ADD.

Common Symptoms of Adult ADHD/ADD:

Difficulty Concentrating and Focusing on Tasks at Hand

Adults suffering from ADHD/ADD often have trouble maintaining their focus on tasks at hand and have difficulty attending to even the simplest daily tasks and responsibilities. If you have ADHD/ADD, you might be easily distracted by irrelevant movement and noise around you, bounce from one activity to another without completing anything, and become bored easily.

It has to be pointed out that symptoms are often overlooked because they do not necessarily disrupt the sufferer's daily activity.

Inattention and difficulty to concentrate symptoms include:

- "Zoning out" without actually realizing that you have, even in the middle of a conversation

- Wandering attention and difficulty to stay on track

- Lack of focus

- Difficulty to complete assigned tasks, even the simplest responsibilities are hard to accomplish

- Failure to remember details, causing errors and/or incomplete projects

- Poor listening skills and have trouble recalling conversations that you were a part of

- Difficulty to follow instructions and simple directions

Tendency to "Over-focus"

Adults with ADHD/ADD may have the tendency to lack focus but they also have the tendency to become too absorbed in certain tasks, especially if they are stimulating. This symptom is referred to as hyper-focus.

Hyper-focus is defined as a coping mechanism for distraction. It is one way of isolating the chaos with an intention of "eliminating" it.

If you have ADHD/ADD, you may have the tendency to become unmindful of everything around you. For instance, you might be watching television and you completely lose track of time that you miss out on what you are supposed to do. Hyper-focus is a symptom that can be rechanneled to increase your productivity but it can also be a drawback on your relationships and work-related responsibilities if the symptom is not managed properly.

Forgetfulness and Inability to Organize

You might feel that your life is in complete chaos and things are always out of control when you are suffering from ADHD/ADD. You might even have trouble keeping track of the things that you need to do daily (even if you are supposed to know your routine already).

The following are the common symptoms:

- Poor organizational skills (evident when you look at your room, your home, your office desk, which are visibly cluttered and messy)
- Easily procrastinates
- Chronic tardiness
- Difficulty starting and finishing tasks and projects
- Often forgetting commitments and appointments
- Missing deadlines and due dates
- Constantly misplacing things, like documents, eyeglasses, keys, phone
- Miscalculating estimated time of completion of particular projects and tasks

Tendency to become impulsive

If you are showing symptoms, you might have trouble inhibiting comments, responses, and behaviors. When you speak your mind, you do not think about the possible consequences of your words and actions. You might be unable to control interrupting someone who is talking, blurting out unnecessary comments, and rushing into working on a task without understanding instructions or directions.

You might easily become impatient. When you are struggling to control your impulses, you might be experiencing these symptoms:

- Poor self-control

- Tendency to interrupt other people

- Tendency to shout out your thoughts that might offend other people

- Tendency to speak or act without considering possible consequences

- Acts spontaneously

- Have trouble behaving socially, like feeling restless during a long meeting

Emotional difficulties

Most adults who have ADHD/ADD find it hard to manage their own feelings, especially when they have to deal with negative emotions, such as frustration and anger. Symptoms include the following:

- Feeling of inadequacy and underachievement

- Easily de-motivated

- Difficulty dealing with frustrations and disappointments

- Is quickly stressed-out

- Extreme mood swings
- Easily irritable
- Cannot take criticisms easily
- Tendency to become short-tempered
- Low self-esteem
- Insecure

Restlessness or hyperactivity

Hyperactive adult have similar symptoms to kids suffering from ADHD/ADD. You might feel highly energetic and always on-the-go, so much that you don't feel tired or exhausted even after completing a number of tasks. However, hyperactivity in adults can be more subtle and restrained.

Common symptoms include:

- Easily agitated
- Risk-taker, sometimes to a fault
- Restlessness
- Easily gets bored
- Difficulty to sit still
- Evident extreme fidgeting
- Constantly craving for excitement and attention

- Talking excessively, often with unrelated thoughts and words

- Tendency to do a lot of things, all at the same time

- Racing thoughts

Hyperactivity is not the sole indicator of ADHD/ADD in adults. You can be less active, yet you can still be suffering from the condition.

Signs and symptoms may be mild to severe, and they may or may not be present all the time. Some sufferers might be able to stay focused more than others. Most ADHD/ADD sufferers always look for something to keep them motivated. They are always looking for stimulation. But there are others that don't need any motivation or stimulation to work on tasks at hand. There are sufferers that can become anti-social, and there are those that tend to become over-social. Their moods, actions, and feelings are often on the extremes.

It is important to be aware of the different impairments that are associated with adult ADHD/ADD, if you want to easily manage and control your condition.

Adults with ADHD/ADD may have these impairments:

School-associated impairments

- Have become underachievers

- Poor performance in school

- Frequently receive reprimands and disciplinary actions

- Repeater
- Dropped out often

<u>Work-related impairments:</u>

- Perform poorly
- Less job satisfaction
- Change employers frequently

<u>Social-related impairments:</u>

- Usually have lower socioeconomic status
- Likely to have a lot of driving violations
- Smoke cigarettes
- Frequently use illegal substances

<u>Relationship-related impairments:</u>

- More marital issues
- Multiple marriages
- Higher divorce and/or separation incidences

Chapter 3:
Causes and Diagnosis of Adult ADHD/ADD

As previously mentioned, about 4% of adults in the US have either diagnosed or undiagnosed ADHD/ADD. This medical condition can have a significant effect on one's quality of life. If you are one of the 4%, you might find it hard to maintain relationships or even keep a job. If you've had the condition since childhood, you might have performed badly in school.

ADHD/ADD can be a lifetime struggle which may cause the one afflicted to have low self-esteem. The quality of life is often difficult and different from most people. When you have ADHD/ADD, you are more likely to have extreme mood swings and personality disorders, if left undiagnosed. However, if ADHD/ADD is properly diagnosed and managed, you'll have a better quality of life.

What are the Causes of ADHD/ADD?

The exact cause of ADHD/ADD is not yet known, despite the continuing research and studies by medical and laboratory experts. Doctors are made to believe that this condition could be possibly caused by structural and chemical differences in the brain. One angle that they are most likely to believe is that a person with ADHD/ADD may lack monoamines, a group of brain chemicals. Their observation that some sufferers are able to manage their condition with medications and treatments suggests that the chemicals in the brain are partially involved in the development of this common behavioral disorder.

There is another theory that genes might be involved, as well, because according to doctors' data, 1/3 of patients with ADHD/ADD have at least one parent that shows similar symptoms. It is also more common if your mother had issues during her pregnancy, including being exposed to medications, drugs, and stress while pregnant.

How is ADHD/ADD diagnosed?

ADHD/ADD symptoms can have similarities with the symptoms of depression and anxiety disorders; hence, getting an accurate diagnosis is imperative. While there is no single test that can determine the presence of the condition, these are what doctors try to include in getting an accurate diagnosis every time a patient comes to them with the obvious symptoms:

- Rule out alcohol addiction or substance abuse that could be causing the symptoms (however, someone who has ADHD/ADD may have alcohol and drug issues)

- Rate current behavior manifestations

- Establish behavior and lifestyle through conducting interviews with people close (family and friends) to the person

- Dig into school report cards (if available) and look for feedback from teachers about behavior problems, like lack of focus in school activities or underachievement

- Establish if the person was diagnosed with ADHD/ADD as a child

- Conduct physical examinations to rule out any medical or neurological illness

- Blood tests

- Conduct EEG (electroencephalograph) tests for abnormalities in the brain wave patterns (this may still be a controversial test, but most doctors attest that it helps them making accurate diagnosis of the condition)

What is the impact of having ADHD/ADD to your life?

If the condition is not treated properly, it might create problems in practically all the areas in your life:

Physical and mental health – The symptoms can contribute to the development of different health problems. These might include substance abuse, eating disorders, chronic stress, depression and anxiety, and low self-esteem. It is also possible to skip doctor's appointments or ignore medical instructions. You might also have the tendency to forget to take vitamins and vital medications.

Financial and work difficulties – Managing finances might be difficult. Many sufferers are always struggling to monitor unpaid bills, tend to incur late fees on mortgages and loans, and may incur debts due to their impulsive use of credit cards. People who are suffering from ADHD/ADD may also experience difficulties and challenges in terms of their careers. There is a strong sense of underachievement within these people, too. They also have difficulty keeping their jobs, following office rules and procedures, sticking to the regular 9-to-5 job schedule, and meeting due dates and deadlines.

Relationship problems – When you have ADHD/ADD, it can put a strain on your relationships, whether family, intimate, friendship, or work. You might easily get frustrated or irritated when your loved ones nag you about getting organized or minimizing clutter at home. You might have a hard time meeting deadlines resulting in your boss becoming disappointed in you. Your "irresponsibility" might be catching the ire of your co-workers and they might even feel resentment towards you.

Having ADHD/ADD can lead to embarrassments, disappointments, frustrations, and eventual loss of confidence. You'll feel like it will be hard to take control over your life again. This is the reason why an accurate diagnosis of ADHD/ADD is very important because it allows for proper treatment.

It is important that you understand everything that you need to know about the condition.

When to Seek Help

If symptoms are hindering your ability to live normally, even if you put in a lot of effort to manage the condition, it might be time to consult a doctor. You can benefit from the different treatments and medications.

These people can help you get accurate diagnosis and proper treatment.

Chapter 4:
What are the Treatments for ADHD/ADD?

If you are struggling with ADHD/ADD, there are a variety of treatments that can help. Treatment doesn't even have to be drug or medications or going to the doctor. There are things that you can do yourself to help ease the symptoms. You may also seek professional help, but in the end, as this is a behavioral condition, you will still have to stay in charge of yourself.

Medications

Medications are not necessarily aimed to cure adult ADHD/ADD; they are to be used as tools in minimizing the symptoms. It is important to understand that drugs or pills won't work for everyone with ADHD/ADD; and if they do work, still, not all symptoms will be completely eliminated. While the popular drugs and pills help improve one's concentration and attention, other symptoms, like forgetfulness, procrastination, poor time management, and disorganization still remain, and these are some of the main problems that you need to address when you have ADHD/ADD.

What You Need to Know

- Medications are more effective when combined with other treatments.

- Each patient will respond differently to any type of treatment and/or medication. Because of this, finding the medication that is right for you can take a little more time.

- While you are on medication, you have to be closely monitored. You have to work with your doctor to monitor the good and bad effects. You have to observe how you react to the medication so the doctor can adjust the dosage if there is a need to.

- Medication need not be permanent. If this doesn't make you feel better, you can consult with your doctor on how you can taper off from taking the pills or drugs.

Regular Exercise is an Effective Treatment

Regular exercise is one of the easiest and considered to be one of the most effective tools in reducing the symptoms of ADHD/ADD. It helps improve memory, concentration, and motivation. Physical activity also helps boost dopamine, norepinephrine, and serotonin levels in the brain. These hormones help you maintain your attention and focus. The good thing about exercise is that you don't need to get a doctor's prescription for it (unless you have other conditions that might prevent you from performing strenuous physical activity).

- You don't even have to regularly go to the gym. A daily 30-minute walk outdoors at least 4 times a week can result in huge improvements.

- Choose an activity that you enjoy and stick with it. Pick activities that will improve your physical strength, or things that are challenging but still fun to do. You don't need to be the best at something, but it's important that whatever you choose as a form of exercise does not bore you.

- There are studies that show that spending time outdoors, particularly where you can appreciate nature and wild life is good for someone who has adult ADHD/ADD. You can incorporate physical activities with exploring nature. You can try hiking or trail running to a nearby scenic area. You can also do your daily walks in a local park.

Sleep is Essential

One of the chief complaints of people with adult ADHD/ADD is having trouble sleeping. The most common issues are:

- Unable to sleep at night, your thoughts keep you awake.

- Restlessness. You might be tossing and turning in bed most of the time and you are woken up with the tiniest of noise.

- Difficulty in waking up in the morning. This can be a daily struggle and once awake, you might feel irritable.

When you don't get enough sleep, the symptoms can get worse, hence, you have to maintain a regular sleep schedule.

Tips to Sleep Better

- Set a specific bed time schedule and make sure that you stick with it, and get up the same exact time every morning. Even if you feel tired, you have to get up.

- Make your bedroom conducive to sleeping. Make sure it is completely dark and put away cellular phones, tablets, and other electronic gadgets that could distract you.

- Avoid drinking any caffeinated drink later in the day. It is even better if you remove caffeine completely from your diet.

- Make sure that you turn the TV off, computer/laptop, smart phone, tablet, etc. at least one to two hours before going to bed. This practice gives you some quiet time without facing a bright screen and conditions you to sleep.

- If your prescribed medication keeps you awake at night, take it up with your doctor to give you a lower dosage.

When You Eat Right, You Regulate the Symptoms

When it comes to *eating right* to alleviate the symptoms of adult ADHD/ADD, it is more a case of *how you eat rather than what you eat*. Most of the time, you might find yourself impulsively eating too much unhealthy fast foods or snacks. These might help:

- Schedule regular meals and snacks of no more than 3 hours apart. You don't want to practice erratic eating because it may trigger the emotional and physical symptoms.

- Consider a multivitamin that contains iron, magnesium, and zinc.

- Protein and complex carbohydrates are important to help you stay alert yet help decrease hyperactivity.

- Eat more foods with omega-3 fatty acids to help improve mental focus. Salmon, sardines, tuna, and some fortified milk products and eggs are rich in omega-3 fatty acids.

Practice Relaxation Techniques

Many symptoms can be alleviated by relaxation techniques:

Meditation – is a form of focused contemplation that the helps relax your mind and body. Meditation helps you center on your inner thoughts. It helps you train yourself to be more focused on any goal you set your sights on.

Yoga – gives you psychological benefits. It teaches you how to perform proper deep breathing and other relaxation techniques to make you more mentally aware. It also helps you cultivate proper balance and stillness.

Therapy

There are health professionals who specialize in the treatment of ADHD/ADD that you can turn to. There are therapies intended to help you manage stress and/or control impulse behaviors. Some of these therapies can help you handle time and money and teach you proper organizational strategies.

Talk Therapy – Most sufferers struggle with longstanding patterns of failures, underachievement, and relationship conflicts. Talk therapy aims to help you deal with this emotional baggage.

Marriage/Family Therapy - This type of therapy will address relationship problems. Part of this therapy is educating your family about your behavioral disorder.

Cognitive-behavioral Therapy – This helps you to identify and eventually change the negative beliefs and behaviors that might have been causing the symptoms. The main purpose of cognitive-behavioral therapy is to change your negative thoughts and behaviors into positive.

Chapter 5:
Living with ADHD/ADD

In the previous chapter, effective treatments were discussed. This chapter gives you tips and strategies that can help you manage the symptoms on your own. When you have ADHD/ADD, you can encounter challenges in every aspect of your life. In this section, you will learn some tricks that can help you manage your condition.

Self-Help Skills to Learn

The following self-help techniques require a lot of patience and a positive attitude. It may be difficult at first but when you begin to reap the benefits, every effort will be worth it.

1. *Learn to Be Organized and Clutter-Free*

Organization can be the biggest challenge you have to face. Your condition can hinder your ability to organize tasks and responsibilities properly, and this can overwhelm you at times.

- Develop a structure for keeping your area clean.

    <u>Create space</u> – Think about what you need every day and make sure that these are the only things that are on your table or visible in your house. Keep the things that you don't usually use in storage boxes or closets. Designate a specific place where to keep your keys, bills, and other items that are usually misplaced, and throw away the things that you don't need.

    <u>A daily planner will help</u> – You can use a daily planner or the calendar in your smart phone or laptop to help you keep track of appointments, commitments, and

deadlines. Take advantage of the automatic reminders on your smart phone and/or laptop.

Have a to-do-list – List down the things you need to accomplish daily, include deadlines.

- Cut down on your paper trail

   Create a filing system - A systematic file will help you keep track of your billing statements, receipts, medical records, etc. Have separate folders for each and label them (or use color-coded folders) for easier identification.

   Check the mail daily – It will only take you a few minutes in the morning to check on the mailbox and bring it inside to check for important letters. Have separate spots for every letter received. You can file them, act on them, or trash them.

   Paperless helps you get more organized – Most utility bills and banks now offer electronic statements, you might want to consider requesting for those instead.

- Properly Manage Your Time

   Time management is a struggle for people with adult ADHD/ADD. You might often miss deadlines, underestimate how much time is needed for a specific task, or procrastinate. You might either lose focus or hyperfocus on tasks that are less important. Here are time management tips to help you:

   Keep tabs on the time – Your wristwatch, desk clock, or a visible wall clock help you keep track of time. Every time you begin with a task, make a mental note or write it down opposite that particular task on your to-do-list.

Consider using a timer – Use a timer or an alarm clock. Set an estimated time of completion and set an alert to inform you when your time is up. For more difficult tasks and projects, set off an alarm at regular intervals. This helps you to become more productive and makes you aware of the time that has lapsed.

Do not rush into tasks – If you feel you need more time for a specific task, set a longer target time of completion.

Plan to be early for appointments – Write down important appointments and make sure to be there at least 15 minutes before the set time. Set up reminders to help you keep track of time. Make sure that you have all the things that you need ahead of time. You don't want to frantically look for your keys or a presentation material when it is time for you to go.

- Learn to Prioritize

Impulse control is a huge struggle if you have adult ADHD/ADD. You might have a tendency to jump off from one task to another, without completing anything.

To overcome this behavior you must:

1. Decide what needs to be done first.

2. Break down large tasks into smaller, manageable tasks.

3. Maintain focus and do not let yourself get sidetracked.

- Learn to Say No

    Often with ADHD/ADD, your impulsiveness gets the better of you because you tend to commit to a lot of projects at the same time or say yes to too many social events and engagements. You have to understand that a full schedule will only leave you overwhelmed and your quality of work will definitely be affected. Learning to say no sometimes is not being rude. You just have to say it politely and make sure that you check your schedule first before committing. This practice will help you accomplish tasks and projects on time and you will be able to manage social dates easily.

2. *Managing Your Finances*

Managing your finances does not only include money management, but also budgeting, planning, and organization. For most people it is a challenge already, more so with adults suffering from ADHD/ADD. Here are some important techniques:

- Take control

    Make an honest assessment of your finances. This will help you gain control on budgeting and money matters. Begin by keeping track of your expenses (no matter how small), for one month. This will help you understand what you are spending on. You might be surprised to find out how much you have been spending on things that don't matter because of impulsive shopping. You can use this to plan for your budget for the following month. Make adjustments on unnecessary spending.

- Create a money management and bill payment system that you can keep up with.

    An easy system that helps you save receipts, important documents, and keep track of your bills is important. Online banking gives a lot of benefits.

    Helpful techniques:

    Use online banking – Signing up for online banking will help you keep track of your balance and other transactions, even on a daily basis. You can also schedule automatic bill payments.

    Set up reminders for due dates – If you still opt to do manual payments, you can make use of electronic reminders.

3. Tips to Maintain Focus and Be Productive at Work

While it can be a challenge to stay on top of all the tasks that you need to complete daily, there are helpful techniques to learn, like the following:

- Get organized.

    Set time for daily organization – Set at least 5 to 10 minutes daily clearing out your desk and organizing paper works and documents. Set a storage space to make your desk clutter-free.

Try color-codes for your files – Color-coding helps you manage and organize your files. It also helps you to easily identify folders, saving you time looking for them.

Prioritize – Identify urgent tasks and put them on top of your list. Set deadlines for all your tasks, even if they are just self-imposed.

- Avoid distractions.

    Minimize outside commotion – You may change the position of your desk so that it faces a wall. You may even hang a "Do Not Disturb" sign to ensure that there are no interruptions as you work. Unless you are waiting for important client calls, put your phone on voice mail and get back to callers later. If noise bothers you, try using noise-cancelling headphones.

- Expand your attention span.

    If you have ADHD/ADD, it can be hard to maintain your focus, especially when you are engaged in activities that do not interest you. Improve focus with these techniques:

    Get topics in writing – If you are attending a workshop, lecture, or meeting that would need your close attention, ask for advance copies of materials, like agenda, outline, or handouts.

    Repeat directions – If you are given verbal instructions, say them out loud to make sure that you have understood them.

<u>Move around</u> – You can prevent restlessness by moving around (but make sure it doesn't disturb others or disrupt the meeting or lecture.

Conclusion

Thank you again for downloading this book!

I hope this book was able to help you learn more about your ADHD through adulthood.

The next step is to put this information to use, and begin working on improving and controlling your ADHD or ADD!

If you are unsure of whether you have ADHD or not, please consult a medical professional as they are the only ones that can make a suitable diagnosis.

I hope this book has been informative, and of some assistance to you!

Finally, if you enjoyed this book, please take the time to share your thoughts and post a review on Amazon. It'd be greatly appreciated!

Thank you and good luck!

Check Out My Other Books Here:

Simply follow the links below to have a look at the other great ADHD books I have available on Amazon!

- ADHD and Children: http://amzn.to/1t18Qc4

- ADHD Diet: http://amzn.to/YgztSi

- Understanding ADHD: http://amzn.to/1ut0cZB

- ADHD and Marriage: http://amzn.to/1pfs64z

www.ingramcontent.com/pod-product-compliance
Lightning Source LLC
LaVergne TN
LVHW021746060526
838200LV00052B/3497